A Perfect Guide To Fighting of Cancer

Understanding, avoiding, and treating our biggest health risk in the best way possible

by

Sarah H. Fredy

COPYRIGHT

Table of content

Introduction

Chapter 1:

      What is cancer?

Chapter 2:

      Cancer survivor

Chapter 3:

      Helping your gut with diet and nutrition

Chapter 4:

      Creating a cancer preventive life

Chapter 5:

      Regular exercise can help alot

Introduction

In the domain of healthcare and wellbeing, few fights are as grueling and emotionally fraught as the struggle against cancer. While medical researchers have worked tirelessly for decades to find a cure for sickness, a potent ally has emerged from the domain of daily decisions: regular exercise and a healthy diet.

These variables of lifestyle have always been linked to better health, but their importance in preventing and treating cancer is just now being acknowledged. This all-encompassing method recognizes the need for a multi-pronged approach to the prevention and treatment of cancer.

Exercise, previously considered simply as a way of maintaining physical health, has shown itself as a dynamic force in the battle against cancer. Nutrition, the fuel for our bodies, has the power to affect the development of illness. The food we eat, the basic source of our sustenance, may both protect us against cancer and be a potent tool in the fight against it.

From the physical and mental benefits of regular exercise to the significance of balanced nutrition, and from the anti-cancer properties of specific foods to the role of dietary patterns in reducing risk, this guide provides a comprehensive and accessible resource for individuals who seek to arm themselves against cancer.

This resource is a friend in the fight against cancer, whether you're looking for methods to prevent the disease altogether or to supplement conventional therapies. Cancer prevention and treatment may be greatly aided by the lifestyle decisions we make every day in regards to physical activity, dietary intake, and other areas of health and wellness.

Chapter 1:

What is cancer?

Cancer is a collection of illnesses characterized by the transformation of healthy cells into malignant ones, which then proliferate and spread throughout the body.

In the United States, cancer is the second leading killer. However, cancer deaths have decreased significantly during the last two decades. Curing cancer and extending the lives of cancer patients is a result of early diagnosis and cutting-edge therapy. Researchers in the medical field are also trying to find ways to reduce cancer incidence by pinpointing the underlying causes of the disease.

What causes cancer?

There is a hereditary component to cancer. Cancer develops when faulty copies of genes responsible for regulating cell division and growth accumulate in the body and ultimately cause symptoms.

Experts in the medical field believe that hereditary genetic alterations account for between 5 and 12 percent of all malignancies.

Cancer is usually the result of a mutated gene that develops over time. Over time, you might accumulate mutations in your DNA that weren't there at birth. Several variables that raise a person's vulnerability to acquiring cancer have been found by medical experts.

Types of cancer:

Although cancer may spread to other parts of the body, its name will always reflect its original location and the cell type from which it originated. A cancer that develops in the lungs but later travels to the liver is still referred to by its original diagnosis.

There are also several clinical terms used for certain general types of cancer::

- Cancer of the skin or the lining tissues of internal organs is called carcinoma.
- Sarcoma is a malignancy that may affect any connective tissue in the body.
- Leukemia is a malignancy that begins in the bone marrow.
- Both lymphoma and myeloma are forms of immune system cancer.

The most common types of treatment are:

Surgery:

During surgery, doctors attempt to eliminate all traces of the disease. In order to eradicate any remaining cancer cells, surgery is often done in conjunction with other treatments.

Chemotherapy:

Chemotherapy is a highly effective but also very hazardous method of treating cancer that targets quickly proliferating cancer cells. It may reduce the size of a tumor or the total number of cancerous cells in the body, therefore making it less likely that the disease will spread.

Radiation therapy:

In radiation treatment, cancer cells are killed by intense, targeted beams of radiation. In contrast to external beam radiation treatment, which is administered from outside the body, brachytherapy is administered within the body.

Transplantation of bone marrow stem cells:

Bone marrow that has been damaged by illness is given healthy stem cells in this procedure. Stem cells are multipotent cells that have not yet specialized. By performing such transplants, oncologists are able to treat cancer with more potent chemotherapy regimens. The majority of patients with leukemia are treated with a stem cell transplant.

Immunotherapy (biological treatment):

Cancer cells are targeted by the patient's own immune system in immunotherapy. These treatments boost the immune system's ability to identify and eliminate cancer cells by activating the body's natural defenses against them.

Hormone replacement treatment

Hormone treatment works by either removing or blocking hormones that promote the growth of certain malignancies. Hormone-based malignancies, including some forms of breast and prostate cancer, are often treated using this method.

Targeted drug therapy:

Drugs are used in targeted treatments to inhibit the growth and survival of cancer cells by targeting certain molecules. Eligibility for this treatment may be determined by a genetic test. Possible factors include the specific form of cancer you have as well as its molecular and genetic traits.

Clinical trials:

New cancer treatments are tested in clinical trials. This may include using FDA-approved medications in unintended ways for further evaluation of their efficacy. Trying out different medicines is also a possibility. Individuals who have tried conventional therapy without the desired results may find hope in clinical trials. This care may be offered at no cost to you.

The importance of early detection:
When cancer is detected at an early stage, it is said to be detected early. Treatment efficacy may improve, and mortality may be reduced as a result.

Cancer screenings may help detect signs of cancer early. Some common cancer screenings may detect:

Cervical cancer and prostate cancer:
Cervical and prostate cancer tests, for example, may be a standard component of annual checkups.

Lung cancer:
Regular screenings for lung cancer may be recommended for those at high risk.

Skin cancer:
If you have skin problems or are at risk of developing skin cancer, a dermatologist may do a skin cancer screening.

Colorectal cancer:
Colorectal cancer screenings should begin around age 45, according to the American Cancer Society (ACS). Colonoscopies are the standard procedure for these tests. A 2017 assessment of the literature suggests that at-home testing kits may also be able to identify some kinds of colorectal cancer.

How common is cancer?

The American Cancer Society reports that 1 in 2 males and those designated as male at birth (AMAB) will get cancer, whereas 1 in 3 women and those designated as female at birth (AFAB) will be diagnosed with the disease over their lifetimes. More than 16.9 million individuals in the United States have cancer as of 2019. In the United States, the most typical malignancies are:

Breast cancer:

Cancer of the breast is the most frequent form of the disease. Women and AFAB people are particularly vulnerable. However, males and individuals of the AMAB make up roughly 1% of all incidences of breast cancer.

Lung cancer:

Second only to skin cancer in frequency is lung cancer. Non-small-cell lung cancer and small-cell lung cancer are the two main subtypes of lung cancer.

Prostate cancer

One in nine men and people with AMAB will get this malignancy.

Colorectal cancer:

Different sections of the digestive tract are affected by colon cancer and rectal cancer.

Blood cancers:

The two most frequent types of blood cancer are leukemia and lymphoma.

Who gets cancer and why?:

Cancer may affect anyone, but statistics suggest that it occurs more often in certain racial and gender groups. The cancer annual report for 2022 states that cancer is:

- More males and those with AMAB are affected than women and those with AFAB.
- Black males are disproportionately impacted by this issue (AMAB).
- American Indian and Alaska Native women are disproportionately impacted by the disease (AFAB).
- Cancer may strike at any age, although the average patient is sixty or older.

What are cancer symptoms?

Cancer is a very intricate illness. Cancer often causes no noticeable symptoms for quite some time. Sometimes the signs of cancer are subtle at first but rapidly worsen. Cancer shares symptoms with many different diseases. Experiencing certain symptoms is not diagnostic of cancer. If you see a change in your body that has persisted for more than two weeks, it's best to consult a doctor.

The first warning signs of cancer are:

Cancer's early warning signs often include:

- Unexpected shedding of pounds
- Chronic fatigue.
- Persistent ache
- Nighttime-recurring fever
- Moles that grow or shrink, or new moles altogether, are the most noticeable kind of skin alteration.

When cancer goes untreated, it may develop other symptoms, such as:

- The tendency to bruise or bleed readily
- Persistent growths under the skin
- Constricted airway
- Lack of ability to swallow

How does cancer grow and spread?

Abnormal cell division:

The body's healthy cells naturally multiply and expand. The different types of cells have different lifespans. When old cells die or become damaged, new ones grow to take their place. Cancer is a disease that impairs normal cell growth. Mutations in the DNA of the cell are to blame.

The DNA in every cell contains instructions on how to develop and divide. DNA mutations are common, but cells can generally fix them. A cell may grow malignant if its error isn't fixed.

Mutations may prevent the death of cells that should be replaced and promote the production of new cells at inappropriate times. These rogue cells have the potential to proliferate uncontrollably and give rise to malignancies.

Creation of tumors:

Depending on their location, tumors may pose a variety of health risks.

Tumors may be benign or malignant. Benign tumors are those that aren't malignant and won't invade other organs.

However, tumors may grow too big, causing complications when they push on nearby organs and tissue. Malignant tumors are malignant and have the potential to metastasize.

Metastasis:

It is possible for cancer cells to travel to other parts of the body via the circulatory and lymphatic systems. This phenomenon is known as metastasis. Metastatic cancers are more severe than ones that have not spread. Cancers that have spread to other parts of the body are called metastatic cancers.

Treatment:

Depending on the kind and stage of cancer, several treatments may be considered.

Localized treatment:

Surgery and radiation therapy that are focused on the affected region alone are examples of localized therapies.

Systemic treatment:

Chemotherapy, targeted therapy, and immunotherapy are all examples of systemic pharmacological therapies that may have far-reaching effects.

Palliative care:

Palliative care entails alleviating health problems connected with cancer, such as difficulties breathing and discomfort.

In order to eliminate or kill as many cancer cells as possible, doctors may often combine therapies.

How can I reduce my risk of developing cancer?

Modifying several aspects of your routine might help lower your risk:

- Don't give up if you're a smoker or tobacco user. Consult your doctor about available smoking cessation programs.

- Eat a balanced, nutritious diet. Consult your doctor for dietary advice and weight management programs if you need assistance keeping your weight in check.
- Participate in regular physical activity.
- Exercise may strengthen the immune system, making it more effective in warding off cancer.
- Stay away from asbestos, radon, and insecticides, among other hazards.
- Wear sunscreen to prevent sunburn.
- Get checked for cancer often.

How do healthcare providers diagnose cancer?

Healthcare practitioners begin a cancer diagnosis by completing a full physical examination. They will inquire about your symptoms. They could inquire about your health background at home. The following further evaluations are possible:

- Clinical hematology and chemistry
- Diagnostic imaging
- Biopsies
- Tests of the blood

Blood tests for cancer may include:

Absolute neutrophil count (ANC):

A complete blood cell count (CBC) evaluates the number and types of cells in your blood.

Tumor markers:

Cancer cells, or normal cells in reaction to cancer cells, secrete chemicals known as tumor markers.

Blood protein tests:

Electrophoresis is the method of choice for clinicians for determining immunoglobulin concentrations. When confronted by certain malignancies, your immune system produces immunoglobulins as a response.

Circulating tumor cell tests:
Cell loss is a possible symptom of cancer. By following tumor cells, doctors can keep tabs on the disease's progression.

Imaging tests:
Diagnostic imaging techniques may involve:

CT scan (computed tomography):
Cancerous tumors' location and effects on your organs and bones may be assessed using a CT scan.

X-rays:
To make pictures of your bones and soft tissues, X-rays require just a small quantity of radiation.

Positron emission test (PET) scan:
Organ and tissue function may be seen using PET scans. This test has the potential to help doctors catch cancer in its earliest stages.

Ultrasound:
Ultrasound imaging employs high-frequency sound waves to provide clear images of inside organs and other tissues.

Magnetic resonance imaging (MRI):

MRIs produce pictures of inside body structures and organs using a powerful magnet, radio waves, and a computer.

Meta-iodobenzylguanidine (MIGB)

sometimes known as iodine.

Carcinoid tumors and neuroblastoma may also be detected with this nuclear imaging test.

The use of genetic testing:

Cancer may be caused by a change in only one gene, or it can affect many genes at once. Scientists have identified over 400 genes that contribute to cancer. A higher cancer risk may be present in those who receive certain genes from their parents. If you have a family history of cancer, your doctor may suggest genetic testing. Cancer patients may also undergo genetic testing in order to get targeted treatment. They arrive at a diagnosis based on the outcomes of the tests. Your diagnosis will be given a stage or number. A higher index indicates further cancer dissemination.

How is cancer stage determined?:

Oncologists and other medical professionals utilize staging systems to assess cancer and choose the best course of therapy. When it comes to cancer staging, TNM is the gold standard. The letter "T" denotes a primary tumor. If the tumor has gone to your lymph nodes, indicated by the letter N, it means the cancer has metastasized. Cancer metastasis is indicated by the letter "M."

The four phases of cancer are as follows:

There are typically four distinct cancer stages. Several criteria, such as tumor size and location, are used to establish the precise stage:

The First Step:

Cancer has not spread to lymph nodes or other tissues and is confined to one region.

Second step:

It's progressed, but the cancer hasn't metastasized.

Third step:

The tumor has progressed and may have metastasized to lymph nodes or other organs.

Four step:

You now have cancer in various parts of your body. Metastatic cancer, sometimes called advanced cancer, describes this state.

Even though stages 1-4 account for the vast majority of cases, stage 0 does exist. Cancers that have not spread beyond their original site are said to be at this initial stage. Most doctors believe cancers of Stage 0 to be precancerous and hence readily curable.

Chapter 2:

Cancer survivor

What is cancer survivorship?

Having cancer automatically makes you a survivor. After receiving a cancer diagnosis, a person is considered a survivor for the rest of their lives. It's not uncommon for cancer survivors to have additional difficulties after treatment.

Cancer that comes back:

Unfortunately, not all malignant cells can be eradicated by therapy. New malignant tumors may form from these cells. Recurrent cancer may manifest in the same location as the initial cancer, in lymph nodes close by, or in organs and tissues remote from the original disease.

Second cancer:

The second cancer is a distinct disease. Second malignancies might arise in the same organ or part of the body as the original cancer, but they are always of a different form. It's possible that they have many forms of cancer. As persons with cancer are surviving longer, they are more likely to get secondary malignancies.

Cancer fatigue:

Cancer fatigue is an overpowering sensation of exhaustion that isn't eased by obtaining more rest. Some cancer patients have ongoing weariness even after their therapy has ended.

Cancer pain:

Constant discomfort is a possible long-term adverse effect of several cancer therapies. One study indicated that 39 percent of cancer survivors had persistent discomfort after finishing therapy. One condition where discomfort may linger even after therapy is peripheral neuropathy.

Chemotherapy brain fog:

When cancer or cancer treatment interferes with memory or decision-making, it's called chemo brain. Seventy-five percent of cancer patients report problems with memory, focus, and task completion to their doctors.

What is the difference between a normal cell and a cancerous cell?

Typically, cellular processes are dictated by genes. The guidelines that genes lay down for cells to obey include when to begin and end growth. Cancer cells defy the norms followed by healthy cells:

- The reproduction and division of healthy cells occurs in a methodical way. Cancerous cells divide rapidly and out of control.
- This natural cell death process is called apoptosis. However, cancer cells are immune to such instructions.
- Regular cells in organs don't migrate. All cancer cells have the ability to invade and metastasize.
- Cancerous cells multiply far more rapidly than healthy ones.

How does cancer start in your body?

Mutations in one or more genes cause cancer to develop. Tumors, or groupings of cancerous cells, are the result. It is possible for cancer cells to separate from tumors and spread throughout the body via the lymphatic system or the circulatory system. (Doctors and nurses refer to this as "metastasis.")

If you have a breast tumor and it spreads to your lungs, for instance, you may have trouble breathing. Some forms of cancer of the blood are caused by the proliferation of aberrant blood cells, which originate in the bone marrow. The healthy blood cells are crowded out by the aberrant ones.

Cancer risk factors you can control:

Smoking:

Smoking cigarettes and cigars and using e-cigarettes raises your likelihood of acquiring lung, pancreatic, esophageal, and oral cancer.

Diet:

Many forms of cancer are thought to be linked to a diet heavy in fat and sugar. Not exercising enough also increases your risk of becoming sick.

Environment:

Asbestos, insecticides, and radon are just a few of the environmental contaminants that have been linked to cancer.

Radiation exposure:

Ultraviolet (UV) light from the sun considerably raises your chance of acquiring skin cancer. Over-exposure to radiation therapy might also be a risk factor.

Hormone therapy:

Breast and endometrial cancer risk may be elevated in postmenopausal women and AFAB adults who use hormone replacement treatment.

Biopsies:

A biopsy is a medical technique used to collect cells, tissue, fluid, or growths for microscopic analysis. Different types of biopsies include:

Needle biopsy:

There are several names for this diagnostic procedure. Medical professionals remove cells, fluid, or tissue from worrisome tumors using a tiny hollow needle and syringe. Lymph node cancer, breast cancer, and thyroid cancer are all diagnosed often with needle biopsies.

Skin biopsy:

In order to diagnose skin cancer, a little piece of skin has to be removed.

Bone marrow biopsy:

A healthcare professional may take a tiny amount of bone marrow for testing to look for diseases or cancer.

Endoscopic or laparoscopic biopsy:

An endoscope or laparoscope is used to do these biopsies. Both of these techniques involve making a tiny incision in your skin and inserting a tool. A thin, flexible tube with a camera at the end and a cutting instrument for retrieving your sample is called an endoscope. The laparoscope is a variant on the traditional scope.

Excisional or incisional biopsy:

Open biopsies include a surgical incision through which a surgeon removes all or part of a tumor for analysis and possible treatment.

Perioperative biopsy:

A frozen section biopsy is one possible name for this examination. This biopsy is performed at the same time as another operation. We'll take a sample of your tissue straight immediately to analyze it. The process will provide results quickly, allowing for prompt treatment if necessary.

How do healthcare providers treat cancer?

Depending on the specifics of your case, your healthcare professional may use a combination of therapies. Treatments often used for cancer include:

Chemotherapy:

Chemotherapy is widely used in the treatment of cancer. It employs powerful medications to kill off malignant tissue. Chemotherapy may be either orally or intravenously (by inserting a needle into a vein). It's possible that doctors may target the damaged region with chemotherapy.

Radiation therapy:

High levels of radiation are used in this therapy to eradicate cancer cells. Radiation treatment and chemotherapy may be used together at your doctor's discretion.

Surgery:

If the cancer hasn't spread, surgical removal of the tumor is an option. Your doctor may advise you to participate in treatment. Surgery is followed by chemotherapy or radiation to kill any remaining cancer cells or to reduce the tumor so that it may be removed more easily.

Hormone therapy:

Hormones that inhibit the growth of cancer are sometimes prescribed by doctors. Prostate cancer patients, especially males and those who were designated male at birth, may be treated with hormones to maintain abnormally low levels of testosterone (a known carcinogen).

Biological response modifier therapy:

Your immune system will respond better and be more active after receiving this therapy. It does this by influencing the way your body normally functions.

Immunotherapy for cancer:

Immunotherapy is a cancer treatment that uses your immune system to combat the illness. Biological therapy might be used to describe the treatment.

Targeted therapy for cancer:

The genetic alterations or mutations that transform normal cells into cancerous ones are the focus of targeted therapy.

Bone marrow transplant:

This procedure, also known as a stem cell transplant, switches out damaged stem cells with healthy ones. In autologous transplantation, your own stem cells are used. Stem cells from a donor are used in allogeneic transplantation.

Risk factors

Certain risk factors may raise your likelihood of acquiring cancer. These potential dangers include:

- Using tobacco
- excessive use of alcohol
- according to an analysis published in 2017, a diet high in red and processed meat, sugary beverages, salty snacks, starchy meals, and refined carbs, including sugar and processed grains,
- not getting enough exercise
- air pollution exposure
- radiation exposure,

- unprotected time in the sun or other sources of UV light

- H. pylori, HPV, HBV, HCV, HIV, and Epstein-Barr virus (EBV) infections, as well as infectious mononucleosis, are all examples of viral infections.

The chance of acquiring cancer also rises with age. According to the National Cancer Institute (NCI), the risk of having cancer seems to grow until age 70 to 80 and thereafter to decline.

Chapter 3:

Helping your gut with diet and nutrition

The absence of digestive issues is just one benefit of gut health. Supporting and regulating bodily processes and keeping your systems healthy is essential, and enhancing your gut health may lessen gastrointestinal disorders.

The digestive system, or gut, is responsible for breaking down food and distributing its nutrients throughout the body. Your GI tract is also vital in fighting off pathogenic agents and is connected to a healthy immune system, endocrine system and cardiovascular system.

The state of your digestive system may tell you a lot about how your brain is doing. The digestive system has a direct impact on one's state of mind. There is some evidence linking the bacteria in your digestive tract to an increased likelihood of developing depression.

It should come as no surprise that the meals you eat on a regular basis have a significant part in maintaining a healthy digestive tract. In order to learn more about the foods that may have a direct and positive effect on your gut health. Williams suggests eating fermented foods and fiber-rich meals like vegetables and fruit, both of which have minimum processing, while searching for foods that substantially affect gut health. You may classify these gut-friendly foods into two categories: probiotics and prebiotics. I said, "Shall we?"

What Are Probiotics?

Fermented foods include helpful microorganisms known as probiotics. Including probiotic foods in your regular diet is one of the greatest strategies to improve your gut health, according to research published in Cell in 2021. "Sauerkraut, cottage cheese and yogurt with live cultures, kimchi and kombucha are all whole-food sources of probiotics," Williams asserts.

However, Williams argues that there is a gap between perception and reality surrounding probiotics. Probiotics are beneficial microorganisms that naturally occur in the digestive tract. Probiotics are sometimes misunderstood as the OTC vitamins your doctor can provide to mitigate the side effects of an antibiotic. Probiotics, however, are the "good gut bacteria."
The most important thing to remember while buying these items is to do it from the chilled area of your supermarket or market. Many bacteria, both good and harmful, are killed by heat, hence probiotic foods are often kept cold. You should also check the labels for ingredients to be sure you're buying a product with active cultures.

When questioned about supplements, Williams says that although they're probably safe, there's conflicting evidence concerning whether or not they really help. "Because there are thousands, even millions of strains of probiotic bacteria, it's impossible to cover all strains with one supplement; in fact, most only include a few strains," Williams says. "And for a supplement to be truly beneficial, you'd need to know exactly which strains you need in order for it to be effective." To sum up, you should still prioritize obtaining nutrients from entire foods.

Probiotic Foods to Eat:
Williams suggests consuming probiotic foods on a regular basis, if not more often. Consuming these potent probiotic foods regularly may rapidly enhance your digestive health.

Greek Yogurt:

The protein and probiotics in plain, nonfat Greek yogurt are great for keeping your immune system strong.

For a gut-healthy and tasty dinner, try mixing yogurt, which is high in probiotics, with oats, which are rich in prebiotics, and fruit. Check the yogurt's label to be sure it doesn't have a lot of extra sugar added.

Kimchi:

Kimchi, a spicy fermented cabbage dish common in Korean cuisine, is high in gut-friendly probiotic bacteria.

Kimchi's use of cruciferous vegetables means it also contains elements with high antioxidant qualities, which may help prevent some forms of cancer in addition to promoting gastrointestinal health.

Kefir:

Kefir, a fermented dairy beverage, is a healthy alternative to yogurt due to its higher probiotic and protein content. A 2021 review study published in Frontiers in Nutrition reveals that eating kefir may help enhance your gut flora by lowering inflammation and intestinal permeability. There's also evidence from studies like the one published in PharmaNutrition in 2021 that kefir may help lower your risk of cardiovascular disease. The same goes for yogurt; read the label to make sure there isn't too much sugar added.

If you're often on the go in the mornings, try our 3-Ingredient Overnight Berry Muesli.

Kombucha:

A fermented tea beverage, kombucha may be carbonated and flavored with fruit juice, spices, and other additives. There are many different tastes to choose from, making this a convenient method to increase your daily probiotic consumption.

Consumption of kombucha has been shown to reduce the risk of developing obesity-related complications, including high cholesterol and type 2 diabetes, according to research published in Critical Reviews in Food Science and Nutrition in 2021.

Sauerkraut:

Sauerkraut, a cornerstone of German cuisine, is a pickled cabbage dish very similar to the Korean staple of kimchi. Sauerkraut that has been pasteurized and is resting at room temperature on a supermarket shelf is no longer a good source of probiotics. If you want to improve your digestive health, look for sauerkraut in the fridge and check the label to make sure it contains active, living cultures.

Tempeh:

Traditional tempeh is created by pressing fermented soybeans into a cake-like shape and is eaten as a staple dish in Indonesia. Tempeh is one of the most beneficial meals you can add to promote the development of probiotic bacteria in the stomach since it is both a probiotic (from the fermentation) and a prebiotic (from the soybeans).

What Are Prebiotics?

Prebiotics are a form of fiber that is not broken down in the small intestine and instead makes its way to the colon, where it is fermented to provide "food" for probiotic bacteria that promote a healthy digestive tract. Williams says, "The probiotics require food in order to survive. Prebiotics are essentially fuel for probiotics.

In addition to helping keep your digestive tract healthy, eating foods high in fiber may help you feel full for longer, lessen your chance of developing some malignancies, keep your blood sugar levels stable, reduce your cholesterol levels, and even boost your heart health.

Eating a diet rich in vegetables and fruit is the simplest approach to ensure you get enough prebiotics. Most fruits and vegetables contain fiber. According to Williams, "you are probably doing OK with prebiotics if you are getting your five servings of vegetables and fruits every day."

Artichokes:

Inulin, a prebiotic fiber, may be found in abundance in artichokes. Artichokes also aid in bone development, shield the brain, and help maintain healthy blood pressure.

Dragon Fruit:

The advantages of dragon fruit extend beyond its aesthetic value; it is also said to aid with digestive health. Because of its high fiber content, dragon fruit is a great fruit for those who suffer from constipation.

Dragon fruit has a form of fiber that helps bulk the stool and offers a laxative effect without creating diarrhea, according to a 2019 study in rats published in Biomedicine & Pharmacotherapy.

If you're looking for a gorgeous, tasty, and gut-healthy treat, try adding dragon fruit to your morning smoothie.

Garlic:

Garlic acts as a prebiotic, or food for the beneficial bacteria in your stomach, so it puts in extra time to help keep your digestive tract healthy. It helps your immune system by fighting off germs and viruses.

There are dozens of ways you may include garlic to your diet, from delectable melting potatoes to warm casseroles.

Mushrooms:

Mushrooms feature a lot of chemicals that may have therapeutic benefits, and they're also high in prebiotic fiber. A 2021 research published in the Journal of Functional Foods found that eating mushrooms might have beneficial effects on blood sugar, gastrointestinal health, and cancer prevention.

Oats:

One of your usual morning meals might be the first step toward better digestive health. One of the finest prebiotic meals that might have a noticeable effect on gut health right away is oats. The complex carbs, plant-based protein, and fiber in oats make them a great food option for maintaining digestive health.
You should restrict your intake of high-sugar oatmeal for the same reasons you should limit probiotic yogurt. Instead, try making your own plain oatmeal using old-fashioned or steel-cut oats and sweetening it with fresh or dried fruit.

Soybeans:

The health benefits of beans are often praised. In addition to protein, complex carbs, fiber, vitamins, and minerals may be found in these foods. Soybeans and other beans include a unique combination of nutrients that may make them one of the most effective prebiotic food sources for promoting digestive health. Further, a 2021 study published in Molecules indicated that soybeans are one of the best-known sources of prebiotics, favorably improving your gut health.

Other Factors to Impact Your Gut Health:

When it comes to maintaining a healthy digestive tract, it may be just as vital to know what foods to avoid as it is to know what to eat. When it comes to your digestive system, ultra-processed meals, fake foods, sugar, preservatives, and chemicals are all bad news.

Williams says that stress, both mental and physical, is bad for your gut health and that you should work to reduce it. In addition, research like the 2021 review published in Frontiers in Nutrition shows that preserving gut health requires concentrating on a healthy lifestyle, which includes things like moderate-intensity exercise and stress management.

Eat a diverse range of foods:
The hundreds of bacterial species living in your gut each provide a unique function and have unique dietary needs.
A microbiome that is both large and varied is thought to be a healthy one. This is due to the fact that the greater the diversity of bacteria present, the greater the potential for positive effects on human health.
The microbiome may become more varied if one consumes a wide variety of foods.

The standard Western diet is, however, limited in variety and high in fat and sugar. Approximately 12 plant and 5 animal species account for 75% of global food production. But in certain rural areas, people tend to eat a wider variety of plant-based foods.

Studies have demonstrated that this disparity exists because the gut microbiome of individuals living in rural parts of Africa and South America is far more diverse than that of persons living in metropolitan areas of Europe or the United States.
A healthy microbiome may develop when you eat a varied diet high in whole foods.

Eat lots of vegetables, legumes, beans, and fruit:

For a robust microbiome, nothing beats a diet rich in fresh fruits and vegetables.

They contain plenty of indigestible fiber. However, some of the bacteria in your stomach may break down fiber, which in turn increases their numbers.

Fiber is abundant in beans and other legumes.

The following are examples of high-fiber diets that promote healthy gut bacteria:

- raspberries
- artichokes
- peas in a pod
- broccoli
- chickpeas
- lentils
- beans
- whole grains
- bananas
- apples

A diet high in fruits and vegetables has been shown in one study to inhibit the formation of pathogenic microorganisms.

In addition to bananas, studies have indicated that eating apples, artichokes, blueberries, almonds, and pistachios may help boost Bifidobacteria levels in the human gut.

Bifidobacteria are considered beneficial bacteria since they may help reduce intestinal inflammation and increase gut health.

The fiber content of several common produce items is rather high. Beneficial gut bacteria, such as Bifidobacteria, may flourish when fiber is present.

Take in some fermented foods.

Foods that have been fermented have had the carbohydrates they contain metabolized by yeast or bacteria.

Fermented foods include, but are not limited to:

- yogurt
- kimchi
- sauerkraut
- kefir
- kombucha
- tempeh

The beneficial bacteria known as lactobacilli may be found in abundance in many of these foods.

Yogurt eaters tend to have more lactobacilli in their guts, according to studies. This population also has lower levels of the bacterium family Enterobacteriaceae, which has been linked to inflammation and other chronic diseases.

Similarly, a number of studies have indicated that eating yogurt helps enhance gut flora and minimize symptoms of lactose intolerance.

Yogurt may also improve the microbiome's function and makeup.

However, a lot of yogurts, particularly flavored yogurts, have a lot of sugar in them. Yogurt is often prepared using milk and bacterium mixes, sometimes known as "starter cultures." It is recommended that you choose either plain yogurt with no added sugar or flavored yogurt with a low amount of added sugar. To ensure the advantages to your gut health, look for the label that says "contains live, active cultures."

In addition, studies have shown that fermented soybean milk may increase the number of helpful bacteria, such as Bifidobacteria and lactobacilli, while reducing the number of dangerous bacteria. Research suggests that kimchi may also improve the microbiome of the digestive tract.

Consuming fermented foods such as plain yogurt may improve the microbiome by increasing its efficiency and decreasing the number of pathogenic microorganisms.

Eat prebiotic foods:

Prebiotics are meals that feed good bacteria in the stomach, encouraging their population to expand.

They're mostly indigestible fibers or complex carbohydrates. Instead, they are digested by certain gut bacteria and used as energy.

Prebiotics are found naturally in many foods, including fruits, vegetables, and whole grains. Additionally, resistant starch may serve as a prebiotic. This form of starch is not absorbed in the small intestine and instead makes its way to the colon, where it is fermented by bacteria.

Prebiotics have been proven to increase the population of beneficial bacteria, particularly Bifidobacteria, in a number of studies.

People who are overweight may benefit from the use of some prebiotics since they have been demonstrated to lower insulin, triglyceride, and cholesterol levels.

Prebiotics encourage the development of various kinds of helpful bacteria, including bifidobacteria. Prebiotics have been shown to provide health benefits, including lowering insulin, triglyceride, and cholesterol levels, according to some research.

If you can, breastfeed for at least 6 months

A baby's microbiota starts to correctly form at birth. Researchers have found evidence that infants may be exposed to some germs before they are born.

The microbiome of a human newborn is most active during the first two years of life, when it is filled with bifidobacteria that are able to break down the sugars in breast milk.

Numerous studies have revealed that, compared to breastfed babies, formula-fed newborns have a different microbiome that contains fewer Bifidobacteria.

Lower rates of allergies, obesity, and other health problems have been linked to breastfeeding, which may be attributable to changes in the gut flora.

Breastfeeding aids in the development of a balanced microbiome in a newborn, which may provide some protection against future illness.

Eat whole grains:

Whole grains include loads of fiber and nondigestible carbohydrates, such as beta-glucan. These carbohydrates are poorly absorbed in the small intestine but are carried on to the large intestine, where they feed the good bacteria there.

Whole grains have been shown to increase the populations of beneficial bacteria including Bifidobacteria, Lactobacilli, and Bacteroidetes, in the human gut. Fullness, inflammation, and cardiovascular disease risk factors were all lowered by eating whole grains, according to this research.

However, bear in mind that some studies reveals that gluten-containing grains—such as wheat, barley, and rye—may potentially adversely influence gut health by increasing intestinal permeability and inflammation in certain individuals.

While this is especially true for those with celiac disease or a gluten sensitivity, it is unclear whether or not consuming grains containing gluten may also change the gut flora in individuals who are otherwise healthy.

The indigestible carbohydrates included in whole grains are thought to foster the development of good bacteria in the gut microbiome. Alterations to the microbiome of the digestive tract have been linked to metabolic benefits.

Eat a plant-based diet:

Intestinal bacteria that thrive on plant-based diets are distinct to those that thrive on animal-based diets.

A number of studies have demonstrated that vegetarian diets may boost the gut flora, which may be related to their high fiber content.

For example, one small 2013 study indicated that a vegetarian diet was linked to lower levels of disease-causing bacteria in patients with obesity, as well as decreases in body weight, inflammation, and cholesterol levels.

According to a 2019 analysis, eating more plant-based meals may improve gut health by increasing the number of good bacteria and decreasing the number of dangerous strains of bacteria.

It is not known, however, whether the positive effects of a vegetarian diet on the gut flora are solely attributable to a reduction in meat consumption.

The microbiota may benefit from vegetarian and vegan diets. However, it is not known whether or whether the benefits of these diets are solely attributable to a reduction in meat consumption.

Eat foods rich in polyphenols:

In addition to lowering blood pressure, inflammation, cholesterol, and oxidative stress, polyphenols have many other positive health effects.

Polyphenols may be difficult for human cells to break down. Most polyphenols are poorly absorbed and end up in the colon, where they are broken down by bacteria.

Here are some examples of polyphenol-rich foods:
- Dark chocolate with cocoa
- Dark wine
- Skins of Grapes
- a cup of green tea
- almonds
- onions
- blueberries
- broccoli

Cocoa polyphenols have been shown to improve human gut microbiota by increasing Bifidobacteria and lactobacilli while decreasing Clostridia.

Red wine polyphenols, which are responsible for these benefits, have even been proven to promote good bacteria in persons with metabolic syndrome.

While human cells are unable to effectively absorb polyphenols, the gut bacteria are able to do so. They may enhance numerous health outcomes linked to heart disease and inflammation.

Increase your intake of probiotics:

When taken, probiotics are living microorganisms (often bacteria) that contribute to improved health.

In most people, probiotics won't colonize the intestines long-term. However, they may improve health by altering the microbiome's general makeup and bolstering the metabolism.

Probiotics have little impact on the gut microbiome makeup of healthy people, according to a meta-analysis of seven studies. However, probiotics may help the gut microbiota in people with certain disorders, according to some research.

In one analysis of 63 papers, researchers discovered contradictory evidence on probiotics' ability to affect the microbiome. The largest impacts of the probiotics were noticed by the researchers to be in reestablishing a healthy microbiome after it had been damaged.

However, some research has shown that probiotics may enhance the activity of some gut bacteria and the production of certain molecules.

Consuming more fermented foods like kimchi, kefir, sauerkraut, and yogurt is one way to enhance your probiotic consumption.

As an alternative, you may try taking a probiotic. However, if you are on any other drugs or have any preexisting health issues, see your doctor before beginning supplements.

In healthy people, probiotics do not cause any major changes in the microbiome. However, they may aid in restoring a healthy microbiome and enhancing its function in people with certain diseases.

The bacteria that live in your digestive tract play an essential role in your overall health.

Numerous studies have now shown that alterations to one's microbiome may result in a variety of chronic illnesses.

Eating a variety of fresh, complete foods, especially those derived from plants like fruits, vegetables, legumes, beans, and whole grains, is the greatest way to keep your microbiome in good shape.

Chapter 4:

Creating a cancer preventive life

Healthful activities may go a long way toward improving your health and decreasing your risk of several cancers - as well as heart disease, stroke, diabetes, and osteoporosis. And don't underestimate the power of a nuanced tweak.

Get your health under control, and get your loved ones to do the same. Pick only one or two habits to change initially. Learn those first, then go on to the others.

Maintain A Healthy Weight:

Maintaining a healthy weight provides incredible health advantages, including a reduced chance of cancer. Some basic advice may be of assistance. If you're already overweight, your first goal should be to maintain your current weight. The value of this alone is undeniable. Then, when you're ready, attempt weight loss to further improve your health.

Tips:

- Make time every day for some kind of exercise or mobility.
- Try to stand more and reduce your time in front of the TV or computer.
- Include plenty of fresh produce and nutritious grains in your daily diet.
- Eat more slowly and reduce your intake of sugary beverages.

Exercise Regularly:

Regular exercise is one of the best things you can do for your health. Finding 30 minutes a day to exercise is a goal that's worth striving for, but it's not always possible. The additional is equal to the superior, but any improvement over zero is welcome.

Tips:

- Do things that make you happy. Exercise may be found in many forms, including walking, gardening, and even dancing.
- Develop a routine where you workout at the same time every day. Take a stroll after supper or to the gym around lunch.
- Exercise with a partner may be a great way to remain motivated and have fun.
- Get out of the house and get moving as a family by visiting a park, taking a hike, or playing some energetic activities.

Stop Using Any Form Of Tobacco

Tobacco usage is linked to several cancers and other health issues. So, don't start smoking again. Quitting smoking or using smokeless tobacco products (such as chewing tobacco, snuff, or snus) is a positive step toward better health. It's challenging, but you can get through it!

Tips:

- Keep at it! It usually takes a few tries to finally give up an unhealthy habit.
- Consultation with a medical professional may double your chances of success by two.
- For assistance, please call 800-QUIT-NOW (866-QUIT-YES in Illinois) or go to smokefree.gov.
- Warn your young ones about the hazards of tobacco use in all its forms. The finest example to set for children is a life free of tobacco use.

Maintain a balanced diet:

The fundamentals of a healthy diet are easy to grasp. Diets high in red meat and processed meat should focus on eating more fruits, vegetables, and whole grains. It's also essential to limit your intake of unhealthy fats (saturated and trans) while increasing your consumption of polyunsaturated and monounsaturated alternatives.

Tips:

- Include fresh produce in your daily diet. Put fruit on your cereal. Eat veggies as a snack.
- Opt for poultry, fish, or legumes instead of pork, beef, or processed meat.
- Replace sugary cereal and white bread with whole-grain options.
- Pick meals that use olive or canola oil, two oils that are packed with beneficial monounsaturated fats.
- Avoid eating as many cookies and other store-bought treats.
- Although a balanced diet is preferable, those who consistently fall short could benefit from taking a multivitamin.

Consume no alcohol if possible.

Six distinct kinds of cancer have been linked to alcohol use. Breast and colon cancer risk is also increased by as little as half to one drink per day. Consuming no alcohol at all is the best option, while moderate drinking may be beneficial for the heart in older people.

Tips:

- Drink non-alcoholic drinks during social gatherings.
- Don't go to any parties where alcohol will be served.
- If you think you may have an alcohol issue, it's important to talk to a doctor.
- Talk to kids about the risks of substance abuse when it's age-appropriate to do so.

Protect Yourself from the Sun And Avoid Tanning Beds

The warm sun feels wonderful, but prolonged exposure to it increases the risk of developing skin cancer, including melanoma. Tanning beds, however, may be just as dangerous. Children are particularly vulnerable to skin damage since it begins in infancy.

Tips:

- Avoid being out in the sun between the hours of 10 a.m. and 4 p.m. It's your best line of defense.
- Wear protective clothing and sunscreen with an SPF of at least 30.
- Don't spend any time in a tanning bed or booth.
- Make sure your children are safe first, and set a good example by always using sunscreen and dressing appropriately.

Avoid Contracting STDs by Taking These Precautions

Human papillomavirus (HPV), hepatitis, and HIV are just a few of the STDs that have been linked to cancer. Prevention of certain illnesses may reduce vulnerability. Try to always practice safer sex, which minimizes the danger of having a sexually transmitted virus. It's also crucial that both children and adults adhere to the HPV vaccination schedules they've been given. Vaccinating boys and girls between the ages of 9 and 12 may reduce their risk of developing cancer in adulthood. However, vaccination is safe and effective up to age 45 (but it is only advised up to age 26). Visit cdc.gov/HPV or discuss it with your doctor for additional details.

Tips:

Be sure that the HPV vaccine is part of your child's routine immunization schedule. If you don't have it, you should ask for it.

- Talk to your doctor about receiving the HPV vaccination if you're an adult who hasn't already.
- Ask your parents or look for your vaccination record if you can't remember whether you were vaccinated.
- For additional data on safer sex and general sexual health, check out cdc.gov/sexualhealth.
- Talk to kids about sexual responsibility and safe sexual practices when it's age-appropriate to do so.

Get screening tests:

Several key diagnostic procedures may aid in the early detection of cancer. Some of these screenings detect cancer at an early, more curable stage, while others prevent the disease altogether.

Screening is recommended beginning at these ages; discuss this with your doctor, since guidelines may vary.

Age 21:

Cancer of the cervix

Age 40:

Cancer of the Breast

- Prostate cancer (explore screening benefits and dangers with a healthcare practitioner for African American men and those at greatest risk)

Age 45:

Colorectal cancer

- Prostate cancer (for men at medium risk, talk to your doctor about the pros and cons of screening with a Medical practitioner)

Age 50:

- Cancer of the lungs (in current or former smokers).

You may want to start being checked for cancer at an earlier age if you have a family history of the disease.

Keep up with your routine screenings and checkups:

Mammograms for breast cancer and stool tests for colon cancer are just two examples of the routine screenings your doctor might arrange. The primary goal of most cancer screenings and checkups is to detect the disease at an early, more treatable, and perhaps curable stage.

Prevent cancer by avoiding carcinogenic substances and other risk factors. Asbestos, benzene, radon, and contaminated water are just a few examples. Be cautious around chemicals like those found in paints, solvents, and insecticides.

Chapter 5:

Regular Exercis can help alot

Studies have shown that maintaining an exercise routine may improve both energy and mood. It may also be linked to a lower risk of chronic diseases and a host of other positive health outcomes.

Any physical activity that challenges your muscles and heart rate enough to cause you to burn calories is considered exercise.

Swimming, running, jogging, walking, and dancing are just a few examples of the various forms of physical exercise available today.

Physical and mental health both benefit from regular exercise. Potentially, it can extend your life.

Learn how your body and mind may benefit from consistent exercise.

Physical activity has been shown to improve mood:

Studies have shown that regular exercise may help alleviate stress, anxiety, and sadness. It causes alterations in brain regions responsible for controlling stress and nervousness. It may also enhance brain sensitivity to the neurotransmitters serotonin and norepinephrine, which decrease symptoms of despair.

Furthermore, exercise may boost endorphin synthesis, which is linked to increased feelings of well-being and less sensitivity to pain.

Surprisingly, it doesn't make a difference how strenuous your exercise routine is. It seems that any kind of physical activity might improve your mood.

Research involving 24 depressed women found that exercise of any intensity substantially reduced depressive symptoms.

The decision to exercise (or not) has profound consequences on mood, even over very short time frames.

One assessment of 19 studies indicated that active adults who quit exercising regularly reported substantial increases in symptoms of despair and anxiety, even after just a few weeks.

Regular exercise has been shown to boost mood, ease stress, and lessen the effects of sadness and anxiety.

Losing weight with the aid of exercise:

Some studies have indicated that inactivity is a key contributor in weight gain and obesity.

Learning how exercise affects energy expenditure (spending) is crucial for comprehending exercise's impact on weight loss.

The three main ways your body uses energy are:

- food digestion
- Exercise
- keeping your organs running, such as your heart and lungs

Calorie restriction while dieting might slow metabolism and potentially halt weight reduction. Regular exercise, on the other hand, has been demonstrated to boost metabolism and hence aid weight loss by increasing calorie expenditure.

Combining aerobic exercise with strength training has been demonstrated to increase fat loss and muscle mass maintenance, which is crucial for both weight reduction and muscle maintenance.

Daily calorie burn and metabolic health are both enhanced by regular exercise. It also helps you maintain your muscle mass and weight.

Exercise strengthens muscles and bones.

Exercising regularly is essential for developing and maintaining robust muscle and bone structure. Weight lifting, when combined with a healthy protein diet, may help you gain muscle.

This occurs because hormones are released during exercise that increase amino acid uptake by muscular tissue. This promotes development and lessens the risk of collapse.

As individuals age, they tend to lose muscle mass and function, which may contribute to an increased risk of injury. Maintaining muscular mass and strength as you get older requires consistent physical exercise.

Exercise not only helps prevent osteoporosis in later life, but it also helps improve bone density in earlier years.

Bone density may be increased with high-impact exercise (such as gymnastics or jogging) or unusual-impact sports (such as soccer and basketball), according to several studies.

Regular exercise is essential for healthy muscular and bone development. Possible osteoporosis prevention

Exercise can increase your energy levels:

Exercise may be a great energy enhancer for many individuals, including those with different medical issues.

After 6 weeks of consistent exercise, 36 participants who had previously complained of weariness no longer felt exhausted.

Not to mention, exercise is great for your heart and lungs. Aerobic exercise is beneficial because it increases energy levels by strengthening the heart and lungs.

The more vigorously you move, the more oxygen-rich blood your heart is able to pump to your hard-at-work muscles. When you exercise often, your heart improves its ability to pump oxygen-rich blood to your muscles.
Over time, this aerobic training results in less stress on your lungs, and it takes less energy to execute the same tasks, which is one of the reasons you're less likely to feel short of breath during strenuous exercise.

Exercise has also been demonstrated to improve energy levels in people dealing with various illnesses, such as cancer. Regular exercise might help you feel more energized.
Regular exercise might lessen your chances of developing serious illnesses.
Chronic diseases can arise in people who don't get enough exercise on a daily basis. Insulin sensitivity, cardiovascular health, and body composition may all benefit from a regular exercise routine. It also has the added benefit of lowering blood pressure and cholesterol.

The following chronic health problems may be mitigated or avoided altogether via regular exercise:

Type 2 diabetes:
Aerobic exercise on a regular basis may postpone or prevent the onset of type 2 diabetes. People with type 1 diabetes also benefit greatly from it. Increases in fat-free mass, blood pressure, lean body mass, insulin sensitivity, and glycemic control are only some of the benefits of resistance training for those with type 2 diabetes.

Heart Disease

People with cardiovascular disease may benefit from exercise as a therapeutic therapy for their condition.

Many types of cancer:

Breast, colorectal, endometrial, gallbladder, kidney, lung, liver, ovarian, pancreatic, prostate, thyroid, gastric, and esophageal cancers may all be prevented by regular exercise.

High cholesterol:

Exercise of moderate intensity on a regular basis raises HDL (good) cholesterol and either prevents or reduces LDL (bad) cholesterol.

cholesterol:

The hypothesis that vigorous aerobic exercise is necessary to reduce LDL levels is supported by the available scientific evidence.

Hypertension:

People with hypertension may reduce their resting systolic blood pressure by 7-10 mmHg by engaging in regular aerobic activity.

However, even temporary reductions in physical activity are associated with increased abdominal fat, which in turn may raise the risk of type 2 diabetes and cardiovascular disease.

That's why it's important to keep moving throughout the week to burn calories and lessen the likelihood of getting these diseases.

Regular exercise is a powerful tool for managing weight and warding off chronic illness.

Exercise can help skin health:

Oxidative stress may have negative effects on your skin.

When the body's antioxidant defenses are unable to fully repair cell damage produced by molecules known as free radicals, this is known as oxidative stress. The skin's cellular structure may be compromised as a result.

Even though excessive and strenuous physical activity might contribute to oxidative damage, frequent moderate exercise can actually improve your body's production of natural antioxidants, which help protect cells.

Similarly, exercise has been shown to improve blood flow and create cell changes that slow the visible signs of skin aging.

Regular, moderate exercise has been shown to reduce free radical damage and increase blood flow, both of which are beneficial to skin health and anti-aging.

Exercise can help your brain health and memory:

Exercise helps increase brain function and preserve memory and cognitive abilities. At the most fundamental level, it raises your heart rate, which in turn enhances the delivery of oxygen and nutrients to your brain. Hormones that promote new brain cell proliferation may also be induced by this.

Furthermore, since the brain's function may be impacted by chronic diseases, exercising regularly can have positive effects on the brain.

Aging, along with oxidative stress and inflammation, promotes changes in brain structure and function, making it more vital for older people to engage in regular physical exercise.

Physical activity has been linked to increased volume in the hippocampus, a brain region critical for learning and memory; this may contribute to enhanced cognitive abilities in the elderly.

Finally, research has demonstrated that physical activity helps mitigate brain alterations associated with dementia and Alzheimer's disease.

Regular exercise is beneficial to brain health and memory because it increases blood flow to the brain. It may aid in the preservation of cognitive abilities in the elderly.

Exercise can help with relaxation and sleep quality:

Exercise helps you relax, which in turn leads to better sleep.

Energy depletion (loss) during exercise activates restorative mechanisms during sleep, improving the quality of sleep.

Furthermore, it is believed that the rise in core body temperature associated with exercise aids in the subsequent decrease in temperature experienced during sleep, resulting in a more restful night's rest.

Multiple studies have shown exercise's positive impact on sleep quality.

One meta-analysis of six trials revealed that exercise training programs aided in improving self-reported sleep quality and lowering sleep latency.

Stretching and weight training both enhanced the time it took to go back to sleep after awakening, as well as the length and quality of sleep. In addition, those in the stretching group reported less anxiety.

Furthermore, research seems that older persons, who often suffer from sleep difficulties, might benefit from partaking in regular exercise.

The kind of physical activity you engage in is entirely up to you. Aerobic exercise alone or a combination of aerobic and resistance training seems to have similar effects on sleep quality.

Aerobic exercise or a program that combines aerobic and resistance training on a regular basis may improve sleep quality and give you more energy during the day.

Exercise can reduce pain:

Despite the incapacitating nature of chronic pain, exercise has been shown to alleviate it. In fact, for a long time, doctors advised people with chronic pain to do nothing except rest. Recent research, however, suggests that physical activity might help alleviate chronic pain.

In fact, exercise has been shown in several studies to help patients dealing with chronic pain have less discomfort and a higher quality of life.

Several studies have shown that physical activity is effective in reducing the pain experienced by people with a wide range of health problems, including but not limited to chronic low back pain, fibromyalgia, and chronic soft tissue shoulder dysfunction.

Additionally, physical exercise may help enhance pain tolerance and reduce pain perception.

The discomfort associated with many diseases may be alleviated through regular exercise. In addition, it may help you feel less discomfort.

Physical activity has been linked to an enhanced sexual life.

Exercise can promote a better sexual life

Regular exercise has been shown to increase libido by strengthening the heart, boosting circulation, toning muscles, and enhancing flexibility.

Physical exercise has been shown to increase sexual activity and enhance sexual performance and enjoyment.

Among 405 postmenopausal women, enhanced sexual function and desire were shown to be connected with regular exercise.

Exercise for at least 160 minutes per week over a 6-month period was also shown to substantially enhance erectile function in a meta-analysis of 10 separate trials.

Another study found that regular resistance training for 16 weeks boosted sex desire in people with polycystic ovary syndrome.
Exercising may boost libido and sexual performance in both sexes. The possibility of men developing erectile dysfunction is also reduced.

www.ingramcontent.com/pod-product-compliance
Lightning Source LLC
Chambersburg PA
CBHW080944260726
48661CB00010B/4080